CW01454635

The Mediterranean Diet Cookbook For Male Fertility

Recipes from the Mediterranean for Health and Wellness to Rejuvenate Male Fertility

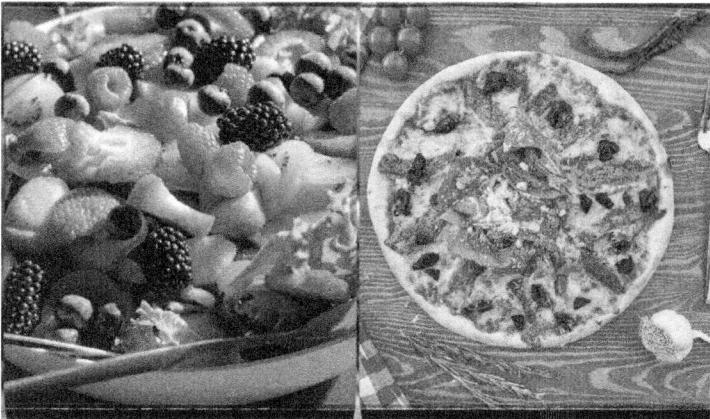

Andrew D. Grady

Copyright © 2023 Andrew D. Grady

All rights reserved. No part of this publication may be reproduced, distributed, or transmitted in any form or by any means, including photocopying, recording, or other electronic or mechanical methods, without the prior written permission of the publisher, except in the case of brief quotations embodied in critical reviews and certain other noncommercial uses permitted by copyright law.

Table Of Contents

.

Conclusion

Introduction

Male fertility is a topic of increasing concern in recent years, as studies have revealed a decline in sperm quality and quantity among men. Various factors, including poor dietary habits, sedentary lifestyles, stress, and exposure to environmental toxins, have been identified as potential contributors to this decline. However, there is encouraging evidence that adopting a healthy diet, specifically the Mediterranean diet, can play a significant role in enhancing male fertility.

In this regard, the Mediterranean diet has garnered considerable attention for its potential benefits not only in promoting overall health but also in specifically addressing male reproductive health. Originating from the Mediterranean region, this dietary pattern emphasizes the consumption of fresh fruits and vegetables, whole grains, lean proteins, legumes, nuts, and seeds. Additionally, it incorporates moderate amounts of fish, poultry, and dairy products, while limiting the intake of red meat and processed foods. Olive oil, rich in monounsaturated fats and antioxidants, is a staple of the Mediterranean diet and is often used as the primary source of dietary fat.

Research has shown that adherence to the Mediterranean diet is associated with various health advantages, including reduced risks of cardiovascular diseases, diabetes, and certain types of cancer. Moreover, studies examining its impact on male fertility have revealed promising results. The abundance of antioxidants, vitamins, minerals, and healthy fats found in the Mediterranean diet may contribute to improved sperm quality, motility, and overall reproductive function.

In light of these findings, there is a growing interest in developing a comprehensive resource that combines the principles of the Mediterranean diet with specific recommendations and recipes tailored to enhance male fertility. A Mediterranean diet cookbook dedicated to male fertility could provide invaluable guidance for men seeking to optimize their reproductive health and increase their chances of conception.

The purpose of this cookbook is to offer a wide array of delicious, nutrient-rich recipes that align with the Mediterranean diet principles while targeting male fertility. By incorporating ingredients known to support reproductive health, such as fresh vegetables, fruits, whole grains, lean proteins, and healthy fats, this cookbook aims to empower men with the knowledge and tools to make positive dietary choices that can potentially enhance their fertility.

Through the exploration of diverse recipes, cooking techniques, and meal plans, men can discover a new approach to their dietary habits—one that is not only enjoyable but also beneficial for their reproductive well-being. By following the Mediterranean diet and incorporating fertility-focused recipes, men can take proactive steps toward improving their fertility potential and overall health.

Basics Of The Mediterranean Diet

What is the Mediterranean Diet?

People who live in nations that border the Mediterranean Sea have long practiced the Mediterranean diet, which is more than simply a diet. The abundance of fruits, vegetables, whole grains, legumes, nuts, and seeds, as well as olive oil as the main source of fat, defines it. The diet also contains small amounts of red meat and sweets, as well as moderate portions of fish, poultry, and dairy items. A comprehensive approach to healthy living, the Mediterranean diet also stresses the need for social connection and physical exercise.

The Mediterranean Diet's Main Ingredients

Plant-based meals, which are a rich source of necessary vitamins, minerals, and antioxidants, are a staple of the Mediterranean diet. Consuming a lot of fruits and vegetables provides a broad range of nutrients and fiber. Because they have more fiber and nutritional value than refined grains, whole grains like whole wheat bread, brown rice, and quinoa are preferred.

The Mediterranean diet places a lot of emphasis on healthy fats, with olive oil serving as the main source. The monounsaturated fats found in olive oil have been linked to increased male fertility. Avocados, nuts, and seeds are additional foods in the diet that provide healthful fats.

The major sources of protein in the Mediterranean diet are modest quantities of fish and fowl. Omega-3 fatty acids are found in fish, especially fatty fish like salmon, sardines, and mackerel. These fatty acids have been related to improved sperm quality and motility. Additionally, significant sources of protein in the Mediterranean diet, legumes such as lentils, chickpeas, and beans also provide fiber and antioxidants.

Yogurt and cheese, which contain calcium and bacteria, are moderately eaten dairy products. Red meat and sweets are restricted since they aren't seen to be necessary for a balanced Mediterranean diet.

Male Fertility Advantages Of The Mediterranean Diet

The possible benefits of the Mediterranean diet on male fertility have garnered attention. According to several studies, following a Mediterranean diet is linked to better sperm quality, a greater sperm count, motility, and morphology.

The high consumption of fruits and vegetables in the diet, which are packed with antioxidants like vitamins C and E, carotenoids, and polyphenols, may help to lower oxidative stress and safeguard the DNA of the sperm. Free radicals, which may lead to oxidative stress and affect sperm function, can be neutralized by antioxidants, which is a critical function.

Consuming good fats has been associated with improved sperm quality and motility, especially monounsaturated fats from olive oil and omega-3 fatty acids from fish. These lipids support the integrity and fluidity of cell membranes, which are essential for sperm activity.

Male fertility may benefit from the Mediterranean diet's focus on healthy grains and high fiber consumption. Foods high in fiber help control blood sugar levels, encourage weight loss, and lower the risk of insulin resistance, which may have an impact on sperm production and reproductive hormones.

Implementing A Mediterranean Diet

Making little but major dietary and lifestyle modifications is required to follow the Mediterranean diet. Here are some doable actions to assist you in making the switch to a Mediterranean diet:

- Increase fruit and vegetable consumption: Aim to eat at least five servings of each per day. To promote a diversified intake of nutrients, provide a range of hues.

- Opt for whole grains: Rather than refined grains, choose whole-grain bread, pasta, rice, and cereal. More fiber and minerals are present in whole grains.

- Use olive oil as your main cooking oil and include sources of good fats like avocados, almonds, and seeds in your meals to replace bad fats. Steer clear of the trans and saturated fats that are included in processed meals and fatty meats.

- Eat fish and poultry regularly: At least twice a week, include fish like salmon, mackerel, and sardines in your diet. Pick skin-free, lean chicken slices, and take off the skin before eating.

- Consume dairy products in moderation, choosing low-fat or Greek yogurt and small quantities of cheese. To get more probiotics, use fermented dairy products.

- Reduce your intake of red meat and processed meats. Limit your use of sugar. Limit desserts, sugary drinks, and other sweets since they don't constitute a large portion of the Mediterranean diet.

- Increase your intake of legumes by adding beans, lentils, and chickpeas to your meals. They are great providers of fiber, antioxidants, and protein.

- Use herbs and spices to flavor your food instead of using too much salt. In addition to enhancing flavor, herbs, and spices provide additional health advantages.

- Maintain your level of physical activity: The Mediterranean diet places a strong emphasis on frequent exercise. Include exercise in your everyday routine to boost fertility and general wellness.

- Practice mindful eating by eating slowly, savoring the tastes, and paying attention to your body's signals of hunger and fullness. Better digestion and healthier meal choices are supported by mindful eating.

You may progressively adopt the Mediterranean diet and benefit from its possible effects on male fertility by following these steps. Consistency is essential since adopting a healthy lifestyle requires a long-term commitment.

Chapter 1: Knowledge Of Male Fertility

Factors Associated With Male Fertility

Male fertility is the ability of a guy to successfully conceive a woman. Male fertility may be impacted by many factors, such as:

- Sperm health: Sperm count, motility, and morphology (shape) are essential elements for successful fertilization. These aberrations all have the potential to affect fertility.

- Hormone balance: Hormones are necessary for sperm growth and function. Hormonal abnormalities in the hormones testosterone, follicle-stimulating hormone

(FSH), and luteinizing hormone (LH) may have an effect on fertility.

- Oxidative stress: Elevated levels of oxidative stress have the potential to harm serum DNA and impair its functionality. Numerous variables, such as a poor diet, environmental contaminants, smoking, and excessive alcohol use, contribute to oxidative stress.

- Swollen scrotal veins are a symptom of the condition varicocele, which may increase testicular warmth and reduce sperm production.

- Chronic diseases and prescription medications: Some chronic diseases, such as diabetes, obesity, and hypertension, may affect male fertility. Additionally, sperm production may be adversely affected by certain antidepressants, chemotherapy, and anabolic steroids.

- Lifestyle factors: Male fertility is known to be negatively impacted by stress, environmental toxins, heavy alcohol, nicotine, and drug use, as well as sedentary behavior.

Dietary Elements That Impact Male Fertility

Because it provides men with the nutrients necessary for good sperm generation, function, and overall reproduction, the diet has a significant influence on male fertility. A diet that is well-balanced and includes the required vitamins, minerals, antioxidants, and healthy fats may have a positive effect on male fertility.

- Nutritional components include zinc, selenium, vitamins C and E, folate, and selenium have an impact on sperm health. While assisting in sperm production, these nutrients enhance sperm motility and morphology and protect from DNA oxidative stress and damage.

- Antioxidants: Antioxidants are essential for protecting sperm from oxidative stress and DNA damage. Fruits, vegetables, nuts, and seeds are examples of foods strong in antioxidants that may increase male fertility by reducing oxidative stress and improving sperm quality.

- Particularly those found in fatty fish like salmon, sardines, and mackerel, omega-3 fatty acids have been associated with improved sperm quality and motility. By including these sources of healthy fats in the diet, male fertility may be enhanced.

- Phytochemicals are bioactive molecules that are present in plant-based diets and have some positive health effects. Lycopene in tomatoes and resveratrol in grapes are two phytochemicals that have been connected to better sperm quality and motility.

- Maintaining a healthy weight is essential for male fertility. Obesity has been related to hormonal imbalances, worse sperm quality, and a greater risk of erectile dysfunction. A balanced diet may help you reach and maintain a healthy weight.

Using The Mediterranean Diet Plan

The Mediterranean diet is a fantastic starting point for improving male fertility since it places a strong emphasis on nutrient-dense, antioxidant-rich, and anti-inflammatory foods. The Mediterranean diet adheres to various nutritional recommendations for boosting male fertility:

- Antioxidant-rich foods: A high intake of antioxidants is guaranteed by the Mediterranean diet's abundance of fruits and vegetables, which may help reduce oxidative stress and protect sperm from damage.

- Good fats: Monounsaturated fats, which are prevalent in olive oil and are a staple of the Mediterranean diet, have been related to improved sperm quality. Additional dietary sources of good fats that enhance reproductive health include avocados, almonds, and seeds.

- Consumption of fish: The Mediterranean diet often includes fish, which provides omega-3 fatty acids. Given that they have been shown to enhance sperm quality and motility, these healthy fats are beneficial for male fertility.

- Whole grains are recommended as part of the Mediterranean diet because of their high fiber content. Adequate fiber intake promotes metabolic health overall, lowers blood sugar levels, and aids in weight management, all of which may increase male fertility.

- Red meat and processed foods are avoided in the Mediterranean diet because they are often associated with poor reproductive outcomes. By limiting particular foods, the diet encourages healthier decisions and decreases any adverse impacts on male fertility.

- Social and lifestyle factors: The Mediterranean diet places a strong emphasis on the importance of social interaction, physical activity, and stress management, all of which enhance overall health and well-being. Regular physical activity and the upkeep of a positive social network may help male fertility.

By adopting a Mediterranean diet pattern, people may boost their nutrient intake, reduce oxidative stress, and foster overall reproductive health. It's important to keep in mind, however, that nutrition cannot guarantee effective reproduction. A healthcare professional should be consulted by those who are experiencing reproductive problems for a complete evaluation and personalized guidance.

Chapter 2: Essential Nutrients For Male Fertility

Antioxidants And Their Importance

Antioxidants play a crucial role in male fertility by combating oxidative stress and protecting sperm cells from damage. The Mediterranean diet, with its abundance of antioxidant-rich foods, provides an ideal foundation for supporting reproductive health.

- One essential antioxidant found in the Mediterranean diet is vitamin C. This vitamin helps reduce oxidative damage to sperm DNA, enhancing sperm quality and viability. Citrus fruits, berries, kiwis, and bell peppers are excellent sources of vitamin C.

- Another vital antioxidant is vitamin E, which protects sperm cell membranes from oxidative stress. Nuts and seeds, such as almonds, sunflower seeds, and hazelnuts, are rich in vitamin E and can be incorporated into the Mediterranean diet for improved fertility outcomes.

- Beta-carotene, a precursor to vitamin A, also acts as an antioxidant and supports male reproductive health. Carrots, sweet potatoes, spinach, and kale are all rich in beta-carotene and can be enjoyed as part of a Mediterranean-inspired meal plan.

- Selenium, a mineral with antioxidant properties, is essential for sperm production and motility. Brazil nuts, seafood, lean meats, and whole grains are all excellent sources of selenium that can be included in the Mediterranean diet for optimal fertility support.

Vitamins And Minerals For Fertility

In addition to antioxidants, various vitamins and minerals play crucial roles in male fertility. These nutrients contribute to the proper functioning of reproductive organs and the production of healthy sperm.

- One such nutrient is zinc, which is involved in testosterone synthesis and sperm development. Oysters, beef, chicken, pumpkin seeds, and lentils are all excellent sources of zinc that can be incorporated into the Mediterranean diet to support male fertility.

- Vitamin D, known as the "sunshine vitamin," is essential for sperm health. It regulates testosterone levels and helps maintain normal semen quality. While sunlight is a natural source of vitamin D, fatty fish like salmon, mackerel, and sardines are also excellent dietary sources.

- B vitamins, including folate (B9), B12, and B6, are important for sperm production and DNA synthesis. Leafy green vegetables, legumes, eggs, and lean meats are all rich in these B vitamins and can be included in the Mediterranean diet to enhance fertility.

Omega-3 Fatty Acids And Fertility

- Omega-3 fatty acids, particularly docosahexaenoic acid (DHA) and eicosapentaenoic acid (EPA), are essential for male fertility. These fatty acids help regulate inflammation, improve blood flow to the reproductive organs, and enhance sperm quality and motility.

- Fatty fish, such as salmon, trout, and sardines, are excellent sources of omega-3 fatty acids. Including these fish in the Mediterranean diet can provide the necessary DHA and EPA for optimal reproductive health.

- For individuals following a vegetarian or vegan Mediterranean diet, plant-based sources of omega-3 fatty acids can be incorporated. Chia seeds, flaxseeds, and walnuts are rich in alpha-linolenic acid (ALA), which can be converted to DHA and EPA in the body to support fertility.

Protein Sources And Their Role

Protein is a fundamental nutrient for male fertility, as it provides the building blocks for sperm production. Including high quality protein sources in the Mediterranean diet is crucial for supporting optimal reproductive function.

- Lean poultry, such as chicken and turkey, is an excellent protein source that can be included in the Mediterranean diet. These lean meats provide essential amino acids that contribute to sperm development and overall reproductive health.

- Fish, another staple of the Mediterranean diet, not only provides omega-3 fatty acids but also serves as an excellent source of protein. Opt for fatty fish like salmon, mackerel, and tuna, as they contain higher levels of omega-3 fatty acids that promote fertility.

- Legumes, including lentils, chickpeas, and beans, are rich in protein and fiber, making them valuable additions to the Mediterranean diet. They offer a plant-based alternative for individuals who prefer a vegetarian or vegan approach to fertility nutrition.

- Nuts and seeds are versatile protein sources that can be easily incorporated into the Mediterranean diet. Almonds, walnuts, pumpkin seeds, and chia seeds provide a combination of protein, healthy fats, and

essential   nutrients,   supporting   both
reproductive health and overall well-being.

By including a variety of protein sources in
the Mediterranean diet, men can ensure
they receive adequate amounts of essential
amino acids for optimal sperm production,
motility, and overall fertility.

Chapter 3: Healthy Sperm With The Mediterranean Diet

Health And Quality Of Sperm

Major determinants of male fertility include sperm health and quality. The Mediterranean diet may increase sperm parameters and overall reproductive performance because of its nutrient-dense meals and healthy dietary components.

The Mediterranean diet's focus on whole, unprocessed foods is a crucial component that favorably influences sperm health. People who follow the Mediterranean diet may lower their consumption of chemicals, preservatives, and bad fats that may have a detrimental influence on sperm quality by avoiding processed and refined meals.

Fruits and vegetables, which are plentiful in the diet, provide vital vitamins, minerals, and antioxidants required for sperm to operate and produce at their best. A variety of minerals, including vitamin C, vitamin E, folate, and beta-carotene, which enhance the health of sperm, are present in these vibrant plant-based meals.

A balanced approach to fats is also encouraged by the Mediterranean diet, which favors good fats over saturated and trans fats. Monounsaturated fats, which are abundant in olive oil and a crucial part of this eating regimen, have been associated with enhanced sperm quality and motility. The advantages for male fertility may be increased by including additional sources of healthy fats such as avocados, almonds, and seeds.

Optimum Sperm Count Foods

Sperm count, sometimes referred to as sperm concentration, is the number of sperm cells found in a particular sample of semen. A sufficient sperm count is necessary for effective fertilization. Several items in the Mediterranean diet may have a good effect on sperm count and raise the likelihood of conception.

The Mediterranean diet is rich in zinc, a mineral that is essential for the generation of sperm. It promotes the growth of healthy sperm cells and aids in maintaining normal testosterone levels. Consuming foods high in zinc, such as oysters, beef, chicken, lentils, pumpkin seeds, and oysters, may help to increase sperm count.

An increased sperm count may also be attributed to diets strong in antioxidants. Antioxidants protect sperm cells from oxidative damage and might boost sperm count overall. Antioxidant-rich berries like strawberries, blueberries, and raspberries may be included in a Mediterranean-inspired diet plan.

Selenium is a different vitamin that helps sperm count. This necessary mineral aids in sperm formation and may boost sperm counts. The Mediterranean diet might contain Brazil nuts, seafood, lean meats, and whole grains as great sources of selenium.

People may increase their sperm count and raise their chances of conceiving a child by concentrating on nutrient-dense diets that include zinc, antioxidants, and selenium.

Dietary Changes To Increase Sperm Motility

The capacity of sperm cells to move swiftly and reach the egg for fertilization is referred to as sperm motility. Numerous nutrients included in the Mediterranean diet may improve sperm motility and increase the likelihood of successful fertilization.

The intake of healthy fats is a crucial component of the Mediterranean diet that favorably affects sperm motility. This diet's mainstay, olive oil, which is high in monounsaturated fats, has been linked to better sperm motility. Avocados, almonds, and seeds are additional Mediterranean diet sources of good fats.

The diet contains plenty of fruits and vegetables, which are important sources of vitamins, minerals, and antioxidants, in addition to healthy fats. These nutrients help to maintain the general health of sperm, including motility. Due to their high concentrations of vitamins C and E, folate, and other vital nutrients, berries, citrus fruits, leafy greens, and cruciferous vegetables are especially helpful in improving sperm motility.

Whole grains including whole wheat, oats, and brown rice are also a staple of the Mediterranean diet. These grains are an excellent source of fiber and B vitamins, such as folate and B12, which support the health and motility of sperm. Adding whole grains to your diet might be a quick and easy method to improve reproductive health.

Additionally, the diet emphasizes consuming lean proteins in moderation, such as chicken, fish, and lentils. These protein sources provide the necessary amino acids that are important for sperm motility and synthesis. The Mediterranean diet may enhance sperm motility if it contains enough lean protein.

Nutritional Modification Of Sperm Morphology

The size, shape, and structure of sperm cells are referred to as sperm morphology. By decreasing the likelihood of successful fertilization, abnormal sperm morphology might impair fertility. Fortunately, there are nutritional elements in the Mediterranean diet that may assist to enhance sperm morphology.

Consuming antioxidants is one important aspect of supporting good sperm morphology. Berries, leafy greens, and colorful vegetables are just a few of the Mediterranean diet's antioxidant-rich foods that help shield sperm cells from oxidative damage and strengthen their structural integrity.

Omega-3 fatty acids, which are emphasized in the diet, also help to improve sperm shape. Salmon, mackerel, and sardines are some examples of fatty seafood that contain these important fatty acids. The form and structure of sperm are enhanced by omega-3 fatty acids, which eventually increase reproductive potential.

Additionally, the Mediterranean diet promotes the intake of natural foods while discouraging the consumption of processed and refined meals. People may avoid potentially dangerous additives and preservatives that can adversely influence sperm morphology by choosing full, unprocessed choices.

The chance of a successful conception may be increased by including a range of nutrient-dense foods from the Mediterranean diet, such as antioxidants, omega-3 fatty acids, and whole foods.

Chapter 4: Recipes From The Mediterranean Diet For Male Fertility

Recipe For Breakfast and Brunch

Parfait of Greek yogurt

Protein, which is necessary for male fertility, is abundant in Greek yogurt. Probiotics, which support a balanced gut microbiota, are also present. The parfait is given antioxidants and vitamins that enhance general health, including reproductive health, by adding fruits like berries to it.

Ingredients:

- *Greek yogurt, one cup*
- *1 teaspoon of honey*

- *1/4 cup of cereal*
- *Strawberries, blueberries, and raspberries totaling 1/4 cup*

Instruction:

1. Greek yogurt, honey, granola, and mixed berries should be arranged in a glass or dish.
2. Till all the ingredients are utilized, keep layering.
3. Enjoy a tasty and wholesome Greek yogurt parfait right now.

Omelet with spinach and feta

Iron and folate, two nutrients critical for male fertility, are found in spinach, a nutrient-dense vegetable. Calcium and protein, both of which are good for reproductive health, are added to the omelet by the feta cheese. The omelet's main ingredient, eggs, is a rich source of protein as well as key vitamins and minerals like zinc and vitamin D that promote male fertility.

Ingredients:

- *Two huge eggs*
- *14 cups chopped fresh spinach*
- *2 tablespoons of feta cheese in crumbles*
- *Pepper and salt as desired*
- *1/9 cup olive oil*

Instruction:

1. Whisk the eggs in a bowl until fully combined.
2. In a non-stick skillet, warm up the olive oil over medium heat.
3. Add the spinach and cook it until it wilts.
4. Making sure the spinach is well covered, pour the beaten eggs into the pan.
5. The feta cheese crumbles should be added on top of the eggs.
6. Flip the omelet when the bottom has set, and cook for one further minute.
7. To taste, add salt and pepper to the food.

8. Fold the omelet in half after transferring it to a dish.

9. Enjoy a filling omelet with spinach and feta served hot.

Mediterranean-style Shakshuka

The ingredients for shakshuka include tomatoes, peppers, onions, and spices. A variety of antioxidants, vitamins, and minerals are provided by the combination of these components, supporting general health and male fertility. Lycopene, an antioxidant found in particular in tomatoes, has been linked to better sperm quality.

Ingredients:

- *Olive oil, two teaspoons*
- *1 chopped tiny onion*
- *1 chopped red bell pepper*
- *2 minced garlic cloves*
- *1 teaspoon of cumin, ground*
- *1 teaspoon of paprika, ground*

- *Cayenne pepper, 1/4 teaspoon (optional)*
- *(400 grams) one can of shredded tomatoes*
- *Four big eggs*
- *Add salt and pepper to taste Garnish with fresh parsley*

Instruction:

1. A big skillet with medium heat is used to heat the olive oil.
2. Add the diced red bell pepper and onion, and cook until softened.
3. Cook for a further minute after adding the minced garlic, cumin, paprika, and cayenne pepper (if preferred).
4. Add salt and pepper to the pan before adding the diced tomatoes.
5. The tomato mixture should be simmered for around 10 minutes or until it slightly thickens.
6. Then, gently break the eggs into each well you've made in the tomato mixture.

7. When the eggs are cooked to the appropriate doneness, around 5 minutes have passed since you covered the pan.

8. Shakshuka in the Mediterranean style should be served hot and garnished with fresh parsley.

Frittata with Mediterranean vegetables

Mediterranean vegetable frittatas contain nutrient-dense vegetables including bell peppers, onions, and tomatoes, much as the spinach and feta omelet does. Antioxidants and vital minerals found in these veggies support reproductive health. Eggs, which provide both protein and minerals that help fertility such as zinc and vitamin D, may be used to make the frittata.

Ingredients:

- *six giant eggs*
- *1 cup of red, yellow, or orange bell peppers, chopped*

- *Chopped zucchini, 1 cup*
- *1 cup halved cherry tomatoes*
- *12 cups finely minced red onion*
- *2 minced garlic cloves*
- *2 teaspoons freshly chopped basil*
- *2 teaspoons freshly chopped parsley*
- *pepper and salt as desired*
- *Olive oil, two teaspoons*

Instructions:

1. Set the oven's temperature to 350°F (175°C).
2. Salt and pepper the eggs and mix them in a big basin.
3. In a pan that may be used in the oven, warm the olive oil.
4. Bell peppers, zucchini, cherry tomatoes, red onion, and garlic should all be sautéed until soft.
5. Over the cooked veggies in the pan, pour the whisked eggs.
6. Cook until the edges begin to set, about a few minutes.

7. Bake the frittata for approximately 15 minutes, or until it is set and brown on top, in the preheated oven.

8. Before serving, top with fresh basil and parsley.

Breakfast Bowl with Quinoa, Greek-style

A high-protein grain called quinoa offers minerals and critical amino acids that are good for male fertility. The nutritional profile of the quinoa is improved with the addition of Greek yogurt, almonds, and fruits by boosting the protein intake and adding vitamins, minerals, and antioxidants.

Ingredients:

- *Cooked quinoa, 1 cup*
- *A half-cup of plain Greek yogurt*
- *1 teaspoon of honey*

- *14 cups of mixed berries, including strawberries, blueberries, and raspberries*
- *1 tablespoon of chopped nuts (pistachios, almonds, or walnuts)*
- *1 tablespoon of flaxseed, ground*

Instructions:

1. Greek yogurt and cooked quinoa should be combined in a dish.
2. Add honey to the mixture and thoroughly whisk.
3.Add ground flaxseed, chopped almonds, and a mixture of berries on top.
4. Serving suggestions: Cool or room temperature.

Toasted Mediterranean Avocado

Avocado is an excellent source of beneficial fats, which are necessary for the generation of hormones. For enduring energy, whole-grain bread offers fiber and complex carbs. Additional antioxidants and nutrients that help male fertility are added by topping dishes with Mediterranean-inspired ingredients like tomatoes, olives, and herbs.

Ingredients:

- *2 toasty pieces of whole-grain bread*
- *1 mature avocado*
- *1 chopped small tomato*
- *One teaspoon of lemon juice*
- *Extra virgin olive oil, 1 tablespoon*
- *Pepper and salt as desired*
- *Optional garnishes: Olives, feta cheese, or fresh parsley or basil*

Instructions:

1. In a bowl, mash the ripe avocado and season with salt, pepper, lemon juice, and olive oil.
2. On the toasted bread pieces, equally, distribute the mashed avocado.
3. Add sliced tomatoes and any other preferred toppings on top

4. Open-faced sandwich to be used.

Recipes For Lunch And Dinner

Mediterranean-style Grilled Chicken Skewers

Male fertility is aided by the required amino acids found in chicken, a lean source of protein. Garlic, lemon, and herbs are some of the Mediterranean characteristics that give this meal taste without adding a lot of salt or unhealthful fats.

Ingredients:

- *2 chunked boneless, skinless chicken breasts*
- *Cut one red bell pepper into squares.*
- *Squares cut from 1 yellow bell pepper*
- *Cut one red onion into squares.*
- *Olive oil, two teaspoons*
- *Lemon juice, two teaspoons*
- *2 minced garlic cloves*
- *Oregano, dry, 1 teaspoon*

- *Pepper and salt as desired*

Instructions:

1. Olive oil, lemon juice, minced garlic, dried oregano, salt, and pepper should all be combined in a bowl.
2. To uniformly coat, add the chicken pieces to the marinade and mix.
3. For the best taste, chill the bowl overnight or at least for one hour.
4. Set the grill's temperature to medium-high.
5. Red onion, yellow bell pepper, red bell pepper, and bits of marinated chicken are alternately threaded onto skewers.
6. When the chicken is cooked through and the veggies are soft, place the skewers on the hot grill and cook for 10 to 12 minutes, flipping once.
7. Before serving, take them from the grill and give them a moment to rest.

8. Serve the tasty and nutritious grilled Mediterranean chicken skewers for lunch or supper.

Salmon baked with herbs and lemon

Omega-3 fatty acids, which are good for sperm quality and reproductive health, are abundant in salmon. Without using hazardous chemicals, the lemon and herbs flavor the food and contribute antioxidants. Salmon is kept moist and helps preserve its nutrition when baked.

Ingredients:

- *2 filets of salmon*
- *Olive oil, two teaspoons*
- *Lemon juice, two teaspoons*
- *2 minced garlic cloves*
- *One tablespoon of dried dill*
- *Pepper and salt as desired*
- *Slices of lemon as a garnish*
- *Garnish with fresh dill*

Instructions :

1. Bake at 375°F (190°C) for 15 minutes using a baking sheet lined with parchment paper.
2. Salmon filets should be put on the prepared baking sheet.
3. Mix the olive oil, lemon juice, minced garlic, dried dill, salt, and pepper in a small bowl.
4. To make sure the salmon fillets are well covered, pour the marinade over them.
5. To enhance flavor, top each fillet with a slice of lemon.
6. Bake for 15 to 20 minutes in a preheated oven, or until the salmon is cooked through and flakes easily.
7. Serve the baked salmon with lemon, herbs, and fresh dill as a filling and delectable main meal.

Olive oil-dressed Greek salad

Fresh vegetables like tomatoes, cucumbers, onions, and bell peppers, which provide a variety of antioxidants, vitamins, and minerals, are often included in Greek salads. Healthy fats are added by the olive oil dressing, while monounsaturated fats and antioxidants are provided by the olives. The entire nutritional composition of the salad benefits male health and fertility.

Ingredients:

- *2 cups greens for a mixed salad*
- *Cuke, one, diced*
- *1 cup halved cherry tomatoes*
- *Thinly sliced red onion, half*
- *Pitted half a cup of Kalamata olives*
- *1/2 cup feta cheese crumbles*
- *Olive oil extra virgin, 2 teaspoons*
- *One teaspoon of lemon juice*
- *Oregano, dry, 1 teaspoon*
- *Pepper and salt as desired*

Instruction:

1. Combine mixed salad greens, diced cucumber, cherry tomatoes, red onion, pitted Kalamata olives, and crumbled feta cheese in a large salad dish.
2. To create the dressing, combine the extra virgin olive oil, lemon juice, dried oregano, salt, and pepper in a small dish.
3. Over the salad components, drizzle the olive oil dressing and gently mix to combine.
4. If necessary, adjust the seasoning.
5. Serve the light and healthful Greek salad as a dish for lunch or supper.

Olive Soup with Lentils

Excellent sources of plant-based protein, fiber, and folate, all of which are crucial for male fertility, may be found in lentils. The Mediterranean-inspired tastes and spices give the soup flavor as well as extra antioxidants and minerals. The nutritious content of the soup is further increased by adding veggies to it.

Ingredients:

- *Dry lentils, 1 cup*
- *1 chopped onion*
- *2 diced carrots*
- *2 diced celery stalks*
- *3 minced garlic cloves*
- *1 can (14 oz.) of veggie broth*
- *4 cups shredded tomatoes*
- *1 teaspoon of cumin, ground*
- *One tablespoon of dried thyme*
- *2 tablespoons of extra virgin olive oil and 1 bay leaf*
- *Pepper and salt as desired*

Instructions:

1. Clean the lentils, then reserve them.
2. Olive oil is heated over medium heat in a big saucepan.
3. When the veggies are cooked, add the onion, carrots, celery, and garlic.
4. Lentils, vegetable broth, diced tomatoes (with juice), cumin, thyme, bay leaf, salt,

and pepper should all be added to the saucepan along with the lentils.

5. The mixture should be brought to a boil before being simmered for 25 to 30 minutes, or until the lentils are done and soft.

6. Before serving, take the bay leaf out.

Mediterranean Bell Peppers Stuffed

The vitamin C found in bell peppers is vital for male fertility. You can make a meal that is well-rounded and has a decent mix of nutrients, including protein, vitamins, and minerals by stuffing them with foods like quinoa, lean protein (such as chicken or turkey), and Mediterranean spices.

Ingredients:

- *4 bell peppers in different hues*
- *Cooked quinoa, 1 cup*
- *Chopped zucchini, 1 cup*
- *Chopped eggplant, 1 cup*
- *Diced tomatoes, 1 cup*
- *1/2 cup feta cheese crumbled*

- *1/4 cup fresh parsley chopped*
- *Olive oil, extra virgin, two teaspoons*
- *One teaspoon of lemon juice*
- *Oregano, dry, 1 teaspoon*
- *Pepper and salt as desired*

Instructions:

1. Set the oven's temperature to 375°F (190°C).
2. The bell peppers' tops should be cut off, and the seeds and membranes should be removed.
3. Prepared quinoa, chopped zucchini, eggplant, tomatoes, feta cheese, parsley, olive oil, lemon juice, dried oregano, salt, and pepper should all be combined in a dish.
4. Place the bell peppers on a baking dish after stuffing them with the quinoa mixture. Bake the bell peppers for 30-35 minutes, or until they are soft and gently browned.

Mediterranean Stir-Fry with Shrimp and Vegetables

Zinc and selenium, which are crucial elements for male fertility, are found in shrimp, a lean source of protein. Vitamins, minerals, and antioxidants are added to shrimp when they are stir-fried with Mediterranean-style veggies like zucchini, tomatoes, and bell peppers. A male fertility diet is supported by the use of healthy cooking oils like olive oil.

Ingredients:

- *1 pound of peeled and deveined shrimp*
- *3 cloves of minced garlic, 1 red bell pepper, 1 yellow bell pepper, 1 zucchini, and 1 cup of cherry tomatoes*
- *Olive oil, extra virgin, two teaspoons*
- *Lemon juice, two teaspoons*
- *Oregano, dry, 1 teaspoon*
- *Pepper and salt as desired*

Instructions:

1. Olive oil should be heated to a medium-high haze in a big skillet.
2. Sauté the minced garlic until fragrant after adding it.
3. When the shrimp are pink and opaque, add them and simmer for a few minutes.
4. The bell peppers, zucchini, and cherry tomatoes should all be added to the skillet.
5. Stir-fry the veggies for 5 to 6 minutes, or until they are crisp-tender.
6. Add salt, pepper, dried oregano, and a drizzle of lemon juice. Combine by tossing.
7. Over a bed of quinoa or whole-grain rice, plate the shrimp and veggie stir-fry while it's still hot.

Recipes For Snacks And Appetizers

Hummus with Roasted Red Peppers

Chickpeas, which are used to make hummus, is a fantastic source of fiber and plant-based protein. Red peppers that have been roasted improve the taste and provide more antioxidants. Zinc and folate, two minerals found in hummus, support male fertility.

Ingredients:

- *1 can (15 ounces) of rinsed and drained chickpeas*
- *1/4 cup drained, roasted red peppers*
- *Tahini, 2 tablespoons*
- *Lemon juice, two teaspoons*
- *2 minced garlic cloves*
- *Olive oil extra virgin, 2 teaspoons*
- *1/8 teaspoon cumin powder*
- *Pepper and salt as desired*
- *Garnishing with fresh parsley*

Instructions:

1. Combine chickpeas, roasted red peppers, tahini, lemon juice, minced garlic, extra

virgin olive oil, ground cumin, salt, and pepper in a food processor.

2. Processing should continue until the mixture is creamy and smooth.

3. If the hummus is overly thick, thin it up with a little water or more lemon juice.

4. Place the hummus with roasted red peppers in a serving dish.

5. Garnish with fresh parsley and extra virgin olive oil.

6. As a tasty and nutritious snack or appetizer, serve the roasted red pepper hummus with pita bread, carrot sticks, or cucumber slices.

Greek-style Filling for Grape Leaves

Dolmades, also known as stuffed grape leaves, often include a filling made of rice, herbs, and sometimes ground meat. The herbs offer flavor and antioxidants, while the rice delivers carbs. The vital elements zinc, folate, and vitamin B6, which are good for male fertility, may be found in this recipe.

Ingredients:

- *1 jar (8 ounces) of washed and drained grape leaves*
- *1 cup of white rice, cooked*
- *14 cups freshly chopped dill*
- *14 cups freshly chopped mint*
- *14 cups finely minced red onion*
- *Lemon juice, two teaspoons*
- *Olive oil extra virgin, 2 teaspoons*
- *Pepper and salt as desired*

Instructions:

1. Cooked white rice, minced fresh dill, minced fresh mint, minced red onion, extra virgin olive oil, salt, and pepper should all be combined in a dish.

2. Lay the grape leaves flat on a clean surface after gently separating them.

3. Each grape leaf should have a little scoop of the rice mixture in the middle.

4. To construct a compact packet, fold the leaf's sides inside and roll firmly.

5. Repeat with the remaining rice and grape leaves.

6. Once the rice is soft and the flavors are well-balanced, place the packed grape leaves in a steamer basket and steam for 20 to 25 minutes.

7. Before serving, take them out of the steamer and let them cool.

Serve the Greek-style filled grape leaves as a tasty and wholesome appetizer or snack.

Skewers of Caprese with Balsamic Glaze

Fresh mozzarella cheese, cherry tomatoes, and basil leaves commonly make up caprese skewers. Protein and calcium are found in mozzarella cheese, while lycopene, an antioxidant linked to better sperm quality, is found in tomatoes. Basil enhances the taste and provides extra antioxidants. Balsamic glaze drizzled over food imparts a tart flavor without overdosing on bad components.

Ingredients:

- *Plum tomatoes*
- *balls of fresh mozzarella*
- *fresh leaves of basil*
- *vinegar glaze*

Instructions :

1. Put a cherry tomato, a fresh mozzarella ball, and a fresh basil leaf on each skewer.
2. Continue until all the ingredients have been utilized.
3. The caprese skewers should be arranged on a serving dish.
4. Apply a balsamic glaze.
5. Serve the caprese skewers as an elegant and straightforward snack or starter that highlights the taste of Mediterranean food.

Mediterranean Roasted Chickpeas

Chickpeas are a wonderful source of protein, fiber, and important minerals like zinc and folate, which improve male fertility. Try making Mediterranean Roasted Chickpeas. When chickpeas are roasted with Mediterranean-inspired spices, the taste is enhanced and a crispy snack or salad garnish is produced. For those on a male-fertility diet, this meal offers a nutrient-rich alternative.

Ingredients:

- *Cooked chickpeas, two cups*
- *Extra virgin olive oil, 1 tablespoon*
- *1 teaspoon of cumin, ground*
- *Smoked paprika, 1 teaspoon*
- *1/2 tsp of garlic powder*
- *1/2 tsp sea salt*
- *To taste, freshly ground black pepper*

Instructions:

1. Set the oven's temperature to 400°F (200°C).

2. The cooked chickpeas should be drained, rinsed, and dried with paper towels.

3. Chickpeas should be well coated in a bowl with olive oil, cumin, smoked paprika, garlic powder, sea salt, and black pepper.

4. On a baking sheet, distribute the chickpeas in a single layer.

5. The chickpeas should be roasted in the preheated oven for around 25 to 30 minutes, regularly shaking the baking sheet to ensure even cooking.

Before serving, let them cool just a little.

Mediterranean Cucumber Cups

Cucumbers are hydrating, low in calories, and rich in vitamins and minerals. Try making Mediterranean cucumber cups. Cucumber cups may be filled with Greek yogurt, sliced veggies, and herbs to make a tasty and wholesome appetizer or snack. Protein, calcium, and probiotics—all of which are good for reproductive health—are added to Greek yogurt.

Ingredients:

- *2 substantial cukes*
- *Greek yogurt, 1/2 cup*
- *1 tablespoon of lemon juice and 2 teaspoons of fresh dill chopped*
- *Diced tomatoes, 1/4 cup*
- *1/4 cup red onion, chopped*
- *Kalamata olives, chopped, two teaspoons*
- *Pepper and salt as desired*

Instructions:

1. Slice the cucumbers into thick rounds, then use a spoon to remove the seeds from the middle of each round to form a cup.
2. Greek yogurt, fresh dill, lemon juice, chopped tomatoes, red onion, and Kalamata olives should all be combined in a dish.
3. Mix thoroughly after adding salt and pepper to taste.
4. The Greek yogurt mixture should be added to each cucumber cup.

5. If desired, add more chopped dill or olives as a garnish.

6. Offer cold.

Mediterranean Bruschetta

Bruschetta is a traditional Mediterranean dish that consists of toasted bread topped with chopped tomatoes, garlic, herbs, and olive oil. Lycopene is present in tomatoes, whereas antioxidants and putative anti-inflammatory properties are present in garlic. Olive oil provides good fats. This appetizer offers a tasty and nutrient-dense choice that is compatible with a diet for male fertility.

Ingredients:

- *4 pieces of crusty bread or whole-grain baguette*
- *2 diced ripe tomatoes*
- *2 minced garlic cloves*
- *Olive oil, extra virgin, two teaspoons*
- *1/4 cup of balsamic vinegar*

- *2 teaspoons freshly chopped basil*
- *Pepper and salt as desired*

Instructions:

1. Set the oven's temperature to 400°F (200°C).
2. Place the bread pieces on a baking pan and softly toast them for 5 to 6 minutes, or until they are crisp, in the preheated oven.
3. Diced tomatoes, minced garlic, olive oil, balsamic vinegar, finely chopped fresh basil, salt, and pepper should all be combined in a bowl. Blend well.
4. Place the toasted bread pieces on top of the tomato mixture.
5. As an appetizer or a snack, serve the bruschetta.

Dessert Recipes

Greek Yogurt Popsicles

Greek Yogurt: Greek yogurt is a good source of protein, which is important for sperm production. It also contains calcium and vitamin D, which are beneficial for overall reproductive health.

Ingredients:

- *1 cup Greek yogurt*
- *1/4 cup honey*
- *1 cup mixed berries (strawberries, blueberries, raspberries)*

Instructions:

1. In a bowl, combine Greek yogurt and honey.
2. Stir until well mixed and smooth.
3. Gently fold in the mixed berries.
4. Pour the mixture into popsicle molds.
5. Insert popsicle sticks into each mold.
6. Place the molds in the freezer and freeze for at least 4 hours or until firm.

7. Remove the Greek yogurt popsicles from the molds and serve them as a refreshing and healthy dessert option.

Olive Oil and Orange Cake

Olive Oil: Olive oil is a key component of the Mediterranean diet, which has been associated with improved fertility in men. Olive oil is rich in monounsaturated fats, which can help reduce inflammation and support healthy sperm development.

Oranges: Oranges are high in vitamin C, an antioxidant that may help improve sperm motility and protect against oxidative stress.

Ingredients:

- *1 1/2 cups all-purpose flour*
- *1 cup granulated sugar*
- *3 large eggs*
- *1/2 cup extra virgin olive oil*
- *1/2 cup fresh orange juice*
- *Zest of 1 orange*
- *1 teaspoon baking powder*

- *1/2 teaspoon baking soda*
- *1/4 teaspoon salt*
- *Powdered sugar for dusting*

Instructions:

1. Preheat the oven to 350°F (175°C) and grease a round cake pan.
2. In a bowl, whisk together all-purpose flour, granulated sugar, baking powder, baking soda, and salt.
3. In a separate bowl, beat the eggs until light and fluffy.
4. Add extra virgin olive oil, fresh orange juice, and orange zest to the beaten eggs.
5. Gradually add the dry ingredients to the wet ingredients, mixing until well combined and smooth.
6. Pour the batter into the greased cake pan.
7. Bake in the preheated oven for about 30-35 minutes, or until a toothpick inserted into the center comes out clean.
8. Remove the cake from the oven and let it cool in the pan for a few minutes.

9. Transfer the cake to a wire rack to cool completely.

10. Once the cake is cooled, dust it with powdered sugar for a decorative touch.

11. Slice and serve the olive oil and orange cake as a delightful and aromatic Mediterranean-inspired dessert.

Fresh Fruit Salad with Mint

Fresh Fruits: Fresh fruits are packed with vitamins, minerals, and antioxidants that can support male fertility. For example, fruits like berries and citrus fruits are high in vitamin C, which has been linked to improved sperm quality.

Ingredients:

- *Assorted fresh fruits (such as watermelon, pineapple, berries, grapes, etc.)*
- *Fresh mint leaves, chopped*
- *1 tablespoon honey (optional)*

Instructions:

1. Wash and prepare the fresh fruits by cutting them into bite-sized pieces.
2. In a large bowl, combine the assorted fruits.
3. Sprinkle the chopped mint leaves over the fruits.
4. If desired, drizzle honey over the fruit salad for added sweetness.
5. Gently toss the fruit salad until well mixed.
6. Let the fruit salad sit in the refrigerator for at least 30 minutes to allow the flavors to meld together.
7. Serve the refreshing and vibrant fresh fruit salad as a light and healthy dessert option.

Mediterranean Honey and Walnut Baklava

Walnuts: Walnuts are a good source of omega-3 fatty acids, which are beneficial for sperm health and motility. They also contain antioxidants that can protect against oxidative stress.

Honey: Honey is a natural sweetener that can be a healthier alternative to refined sugar. It provides antioxidants and may have potential benefits for reproductive health.

Ingredients:

- *1 package phyllo dough*
- *1 cup chopped walnuts*
- *¼ cup honey*
- *2 tablespoons unsalted butter, melted*
- *1 teaspoon ground cinnamon*

Instructions:

1. Preheat the oven to 350°F (175°C).
2. In a bowl, combine the chopped walnuts, honey, melted butter, and ground cinnamon. Mix well.
3. Place one sheet of phyllo dough on a greased baking sheet. Brush it with melted

butter, then add another sheet on top and brush with butter again. Repeat this process until you have used half of the phyllo dough.

4. Spread the walnut mixture evenly over the layered phyllo dough.

5. Continue layering the remaining sheets of phyllo dough, brushing each one with melted butter.

6. Using a sharp knife, cut the baklava into diamond or square shapes.

7. Bake in the preheated oven for about 30-35 minutes or until golden brown.

8. Remove from the oven and allow it to cool before serving.

Mediterranean Yogurt Parfait

Yogurt: Yogurt is a good source of protein and calcium, which are important for sperm production and overall reproductive health. It also contains probiotics that may support gut health, which can indirectly influence fertility.

Ingredients:

- *1 cup Greek yogurt*
- *2 tablespoons honey*
- *¼ cup mixed berries (blueberries, raspberries, strawberries)*
- *2 tablespoons chopped nuts (almonds, walnuts, or pistachios)*
- *1 tablespoon ground flaxseed*

Instructions:

1. In a glass or a bowl, layer Greek yogurt, drizzle honey over it, and top with mixed berries.
2. Sprinkle with chopped nuts and ground flaxseed.
3. Repeat the layers if desired.
4. Serve chilled.

Mediterranean Fruit Sorbet

Fresh Fruits: Similar to the fruit salad, the Mediterranean fruit sorbet provides the nutritional benefits of fresh fruits, including vitamins, minerals, and antioxidants

Ingredients:

- *2 cups frozen mixed berries (blueberries, raspberries, strawberries)*
- *1 ripe banana*
- *2 tablespoons honey*
- *1 tablespoon lemon juice*

Instructions:

1. In a blender or food processor, combine the frozen mixed berries, ripe banana, honey, and lemon juice.
2. Blend until smooth and creamy.
3. If the mixture is too thick, you can add a small amount of water or a splash of fruit juice to help with blending.
4. Transfer the sorbet mixture into a freezer-safe container and freeze for at least 2-3 hours or until firm.
5. Scoop the sorbet into serving bowls and enjoy.

You may reap the advantages of a fertility-enhancing diet while relishing the colorful tastes and health-promoting components of Mediterranean cuisine by including these Mediterranean diet dishes in your everyday meals.

Chapter 5: Mediterranean Diet Meal Plans

Weekly Meal Plan For Male Fertility

We will go into detail about developing a thorough weekly food plan in this chapter that is particularly created to boost male fertility with the Mediterranean diet. People may include a range of nutrient-dense meals that have been linked to better sperm quality and reproductive health by adhering to these meal plans.

Let's look at an example weekly meal plan that focuses on male fertility while including the main ideas of the Mediterranean diet. Please be aware that this program may be modified to accommodate unique tastes and dietary requirements.

Monday:

Breakfast: Greek yogurt topped with mixed berries and a sprinkle of crushed almonds. Serve with whole grain toast.
Snack: A handful of walnuts and an apple.
Lunch: Mediterranean salad with mixed greens, cherry tomatoes, cucumbers, feta cheese, olives, and grilled chicken. Dress with olive oil and lemon juice.
Snack: Carrot sticks with hummus.
Dinner: Baked salmon seasoned with herbs and served with a side of quinoa and roasted vegetables.
Dessert: Fresh fruit salad.

Tuesday:

Breakfast: Omelet made with spinach, tomatoes, and feta cheese. Serve with whole wheat toast.
Snack: Greek yogurt with honey and a handful of almonds.

Lunch: Whole grain pasta with homemade tomato sauce, topped with grilled shrimp and a sprinkle of Parmesan cheese.

Snack: Sliced bell peppers with tzatziki sauce.

Dinner: Grilled chicken breast with a side of roasted sweet potatoes and steamed broccoli.

Dessert: Dark chocolate-covered strawberries.

Wednesday:

Breakfast: Overnight oats made with rolled oats, almond milk, chia seeds, and a topping of mixed nuts and dried fruits.

Snack: Fresh grapes and a small portion of cheese.

Lunch: Quinoa salad with cherry tomatoes, cucumber, red onion, Kalamata olives, and crumbled feta cheese. Dress with olive oil and lemon juice.

Snack: Homemade trail mix with dried fruits and nuts.

Dinner: Baked cod fillet with lemon and herbs, served with a side of whole grain couscous and steamed asparagus.

Dessert: Yogurt with a drizzle of honey and a sprinkle of cinnamon.

Thursday:

Breakfast: Whole grain toast with avocado, tomato slices, and a poached egg.

Snack: A handful of almonds and a banana.

Lunch: Greek salad with romaine lettuce, tomatoes, cucumbers, red onions, feta cheese, and grilled chicken. Dress with olive oil and red wine vinegar.

Snack: Sliced cucumber with tzatziki sauce.

Dinner: Mediterranean-style turkey meatballs served with whole wheat pasta and sautéed zucchini.

Dessert: Fresh mixed berries with a dollop of Greek yogurt.

Friday:

Breakfast: Vegetable frittata made with spinach, bell peppers, onions, and feta cheese.

Snack: Mixed nuts and dried fruits.

Lunch: Lentil soup with a side of whole grain bread.

Snack: Greek yogurt with honey and sliced almonds.

Dinner: Grilled steak with a side of roasted potatoes and steamed green beans.

Dessert: Grilled pineapple slices with a sprinkle of cinnamon.

Saturday:

Breakfast: Whole wheat pancakes topped with fresh berries and a drizzle of maple syrup.

Snack: Carrot sticks with hummus.

Lunch: Mediterranean-style wrap with grilled chicken, tzatziki sauce, mixed greens, tomatoes, and cucumbers.

Snack: Fresh grapes and a small portion of cheese.

Dinner: Baked eggplant Parmesan served with a side of whole grain spaghetti and a green salad.

Dessert: Lemon sorbet.

Sunday:

Breakfast: Smoked salmon and avocado toast on whole grain bread.

Snack: A handful of walnuts and a banana.

Lunch: Grilled shrimp skewers with a side of quinoa salad, including cherry tomatoes, cucumber, red onion, and parsley. Dress with olive oil and lemon juice.

Snack: Greek yogurt with honey and sliced almonds.

Dinner: Mediterranean-style grilled vegetables (such as zucchini, bell peppers, and eggplant) served with grilled chicken breast and a side of whole grain couscous.

Dessert: Mixed fruit skewers with a drizzle of honey.

By following this sample weekly meal plan, individuals can enjoy a diverse range of nutrient-rich foods while adhering to the principles of the Mediterranean diet. The plan includes a balance of lean proteins, whole grains, fruits, vegetables, healthy fats, and low-fat dairy products, all of which have been associated with enhanced male fertility.

Grocery Shopping List

To successfully execute the Mediterranean diet meal plans for male fertility, it's essential to have the right ingredients on hand. Below is a comprehensive grocery shopping list to guide you:

Proteins:

- *Chicken breast*
- *Salmon*
- *Cod filet*
- *Shrimp*
- *Lean beef steak*
- *Turkey meatballs*

- *Eggs*
- *Greek yogurt*
- *Feta cheese*
- *Parmesan cheese*

Whole Grains:

- *Whole wheat bread*
- *Whole grain pasta*
- *Quinoa*
- *Couscous*
- *Rolled oats*

Fruits and Vegetables:

- *Mixed berries (such as strawberries, blueberries, raspberries)*
- *Apples*
- *Oranges*
- *Grapes*
- *Bananas*
- *Avocado*
- *Tomatoes*
- *Cucumbers*

- *Bell peppers*
- *Spinach*
- *Romaine lettuce*
- *Red onions*
- *Asparagus*
- *Broccoli*
- *Sweet potatoes*
- *Zucchini*
- *Eggplant*
- *Parsley*
- *Lemons*
- *Limes*

Healthy Fats and Condiments:

- *Olive oil*
- *Almonds*
- *Walnuts*
- *Mixed nuts*
- *Dried fruits*
- *Hummus*
- *Tzatziki sauce*
- *Honey*
- *Maple syrup*

Other Essentials:

- *Whole grain crackers*
- *Whole wheat pancakes*
- *Lentils*
- *Vegetable broth*
- *Dark chocolate*
- *Cinnamon*
- *Red wine vinegar*

This grocery shopping list provides a solid foundation for creating nutritious meals while following the Mediterranean diet principles and promoting male fertility.

Advice On How To Prepare Meals And Control Portion Size

Take into account the following advice to successfully adopt the Mediterranean diet meal plans and achieve correct quantity control:

- Spend some time each week planning your meals, taking into account the items you have on hand and your dietary preferences. You can remain organized and stop compulsive eating with the aid of this.

- Prepare ingredients ahead of time: Fruits and vegetables should be washed and chopped in advance so that they are accessible for cooking or eating. This will enable you to prepare meals more quickly.

- Cook in bulk: Make bigger servings of certain meals so that you can keep and eat the leftovers. As a result, there is a lesser need for everyday cooking, and meals may be prepared quickly and conveniently throughout the week.

- Use smaller plates: To regulate portion proportions, use smaller plates and bowls. According to research, consumers often consume less food when it is presented on smaller plates.

- Veggies should take up at least half of your plate; try to choose a range of vibrantly colored veggies. This guarantees that you get enough of the important vitamins, minerals, and fiber in your diet.

- Watch your protein intake: When it comes to proteins, watch your portion sizes. Aim for a serving size that is around the size of a deck of cards, or approximately 3 to 4 ounces. This keeps your protein consumption balanced without going overboard.

- Choose healthier cooking techniques: Consider grilling, baking, steaming, or sautéing with little to no oil. Avoid deep-frying or using a lot of oil on your food since this might add extra calories.

- Limit added sugars and processed foods: It's crucial to limit your intake of these items when adhering to the Mediterranean diet. To increase nutritional content, emphasize using whole, unprocessed foods as much as possible.

- Keep hydrated: To maintain appropriate hydration, sip copious amounts of water throughout the day. Limit sugary drinks and use water as your main hydration option.

- Eat slowly and mindfully, paying attention to your body's signals of hunger and fullness with each meal. This encourages a better connection with food and prevents overeating.

- Make the meal plans specific to your needs: You are free to change the example meal plans to suit your dietary needs, food allergies, or other restrictions. To make the meal plans suitable for you, swap out components or change the portion proportions as necessary.

You may successfully stick to the Mediterranean diet meal plans for male fertility by using these guidelines for meal preparation and quantity management. Always pay attention to your body's signals, choose nutritious foods, and take pleasure in the act of feeding yourself good, fertility-boosting meals.

Chapter 6: Male Fertility And The Mediterranean Diet And Lifestyle

To better boost male fertility, this chapter explores the significance of incorporating Mediterranean lifestyle practices into daily routines. It also examines different lifestyle elements, such as exercise, stress reduction, and sufficient sleep, that may have a good influence on reproductive health. You may maximize your fertility and increase the advantages of the Mediterranean diet by adopting these routines into your everyday life.

Male Fertility And Physical Activity

Regular exercise is important for general health and may have a big impact on male fertility. Exercise of moderate intensity has been linked to enhanced hormone balance and sperm quality. Incorporating physical exercise into your Mediterranean lifestyle is suggested by the following:

- Aim for 150 minutes or more per week of aerobic activity at a moderate level. This may involve exercises like running, cycling, swimming, or fast walking.

- To increase muscle growth and general fitness, including strength training activities at least two days a week. Free weights, resistance bands, or bodyweight workouts may be used in this.

- To remain motivated, engage in things you want to do. Think about engaging in group exercise activities, taking dancing lessons, or joining a sports team.

- Include exercise in your everyday regimen. Use the stairs instead of the elevator, go to nearby locations on foot or by bicycle, and indulge in physical activities like gardening or outdoor games.

- Always check with your doctor before beginning a new workout program, particularly if you have any underlying medical issues.

Stress Reduction To Improve Male Fertility

Male fertility might suffer from chronic stress because it alters hormone levels and sperm production. Stress control is crucial for achieving reproductive health optimization. Consider incorporating the following tactics into your Mediterranean way of life:

- Use relaxation methods like yoga, meditation, or deep breathing exercises. These pursuits support general well-being by lowering stress levels.

- Take part in interests and pursuits that make you happy and relieve stress. You may do things like read, paint, listen to music, or spend time in nature.

- Ensure a good work-life balance. Prioritize self-care activities and establish boundaries between your personal and professional lives.

- If stress becomes unbearable, ask for help from loved ones or think about seeking professional therapy.

Sufficient Sleep Promotes Male Fertility

For hormonal balance and reproductive health, quality sleep is essential. Male fertility may suffer as a result of sleep deprivation or poor sleep quality. Here are some pointers for encouraging better sleep:

- By going to bed and getting up at the same time each day, even on the weekends, you may create a regular sleeping routine.

- To tell your body it's time to wind down, establish a calming sleep ritual. This could include doing things like reading, taking a warm bath, or other relaxation methods.

- Maintain a cool, calm, and dark sleeping environment in your bedroom. Use cozy bedding and make sure there is enough airflow.

- Avoid using electronics, consuming coffee, and engaging in stimulating activities just before bed since these things might disrupt your sleep.

Regular physical exercise, appropriate stress management, and enough sleep are essential lifestyle practices that boost male fertility in addition to the Mediterranean diet. You may establish a comprehensive approach to reproductive health and increase the advantages of the Mediterranean diet by including these routines in your everyday life.

Conclusion

It's important to keep in mind that patience and consistency are vital when people start this path to increase their fertility via dietary modifications. Results may not show up right away, so it's critical to maintain your commitment to dietary adjustments that will remain.

It's advised to keep adopting these dietary guidelines and lifestyle practices into everyday living to optimize the Mediterranean diet's advantages for male fertility. Long-term reproductive health will be influenced by consistency in nutrition, quantity management, and adherence to a balanced and nutritious diet.

Here are a few last hints and suggestions to improve the outcomes:

- Maintain current knowledge: Continue to keep up with the most recent findings in the fields of male fertility and the Mediterranean diet. Keep an open mind to new information and modify your diet as necessary.

- Consult a professional: If you have certain health concerns or fertility problems, you may want to speak with a registered dietitian who specializes in reproductive health or a member of the medical profession. They may provide individualized advice and assistance catered to your particular need.

- Exercise restraint and flexibility: While the Mediterranean diet has many health advantages, it's crucial to keep a balanced lifestyle. Give yourself periodic treats, and customize the diet to your tastes and cultural customs.

- Encourage your spouse to follow the Mediterranean diet and lifestyle by including them. You may improve the atmosphere and raise the likelihood of favorable reproductive outcomes by supporting one another.

- Remain upbeat and persistent since boosting fertility and changing eating habits take time. Stay upbeat, acknowledge minor successes, and exercise patience at all times.

You may continue on your path to enhancing male fertility and general reproductive health by putting these suggestions and practices into practice. Always keep in mind that the Mediterranean diet has long-term advantages beyond fertility and is not simply a short-term fix.

I wish you well as you work to improve male fertility and live a better, happier life!

Printed in Great Britain
by Amazon

28705319R00059